WOMAN

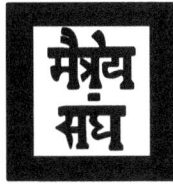

WOMAN

FROM AGNI YOGA TEACHINGS

AGNI YOGA SOCIETY
2019

Agni Yoga Society
319 West 107th Street
New York NY 10025
www.agniyoga.org

Reprinted 2019.

ISBN: 978-0-933574-19-9

Dedicated
to all women who strive
toward the Light of Understanding
for the upliftment of humanity
in the New Era

WOMAN

Selections from the books of the
Agni Yoga Teachings for the New Era

- *Leaves of Morya's Garden I, The Call,* 1924
- *Leaves of Morya's Garden II, Illumination,* 1925
- *New Era Community,* 1926
- *Agni Yoga,* 1929
- *Infinity I,* 1930
- *Infinity II,* 1930
- *Hierarchy,* 1931
- *Heart,* 1932
- *Fiery World I,* 1933
- *Fiery World II,* 1934
- *Fiery World III,* 1935
- *Aum,* 1936
- *Brotherhood*, 1937
- *Letters of Helena Roerich,* 1929-1938, Volume I

FOREWORD (1958)

THE equilibrium of the elements is a foundation of Life, and the violation of this law leads to destruction. And now the Great Teachers will affirm the rights of woman. Therefore, the coming epoch will be not only an epoch of great cooperation, it will also be the Epoch of Woman. Woman will have to be armed with courage, and, first of all, she will have to restrain her heart from unwise giving, for there must be the Golden Balance in everything. Woman must affirm herself, and that is why the Sword of Spirit is given precisely into the hands of woman. In the East this epoch is noted as the Epoch of Maitreya, the Epoch of Great Compassion, and the Epoch of the Mother of the World.

Letters of Helena Roerich,
Vol. I, page 376.

WOMAN

Leaves of Morya's Garden Vol. I, The Call

13. The daughter of the world may vanquish destiny.

The New World approaches—sacrifices are the steps of ascent.

The growth is quickened by faith if the spirit is ready to receive.

345. In ancient cults there always remained vestiges of spiritual teachings.

Even the old choral ring dance retained the principle of spirituality.

In the center of the ring was placed the chosen one— most often a woman.

Around her circled the ritualistic figures of the chorus.

The chosen one in the center remained as if inert.

But all the movements and invocations were as if directed toward her.

And she took upon herself the significance of expression of all aspirations.

Just so is it in the teaching of the Spirit.

The disciple acquires the illumination of joy.

357. They are rending the Raiment of the Lord.

They scoff at its tatters.

But the daughter of the world and the Mother of the Universe will join the pieces of this Raiment.

And thou wilt come ready to receive thy vestment.

For, wherefore the power and wherefore the sacrifice,
if there be no joy?

And where is compassion,

And where is devotion,

And where is the love of creation,

If thy shoulders are not bedecked with the
Raiment of the Mother of the World?

421. Do we trouble the long-awaited visitor with
personal wishes?

We hasten to open the gates so that the desired one
may come in.

Often the hand is outstretched,

But the blind try to reject it.

Therefore, to suppress the conception of children is
worse than murder.

Also, it is not right to pile up a complex of one's own
wishes.

Before the coming of the guest it is better to ventilate
the house, and in quiet, repeating a prayer, to
direct one's eyes to beauty.

Not necessary are countless speculations and
designations—

The spirit proceeds freely.

Earth's burden must be lifted.

Layers of effluvia enwrap every cradle.

Blessed is the mother who draws open the curtain to
let in the light, and who offers the first blossom.

In quiet, in beauty, and with a smile,

Await those new ones seeking entry into the world.

433. The Wonders of the Teacher will grow.

Amidst the garden of love grow illuminations of the spirit.

Tire Me today; burden Me more, laying on the weight of the world.

Yet will I increase My strength.

Yet will I increase the strength of My daughter, for she goes into My garden.

Dost thou hear? The burden will blossom as roses,

And the grass will be arrayed with the morning rainbow.

Therefore, tire Me.

When I go into the beautiful garden I fear no burden.

I ponder, I ponder, I ponder.

449. I will assemble the daughters.

Let them help lay out the beautiful garden.

Let them fill the garden to overflowing with new blossoms.

I perceive that one can expect a rapid sprouting of the life of the New World.

452. When a maiden strives evenings and nights to bring good to the world—

When she dreams about the ineffably beautiful and lofty—is this remote from life?

If these dreams be beautiful, will not the response to them also be beautiful?

Leaves of Marya's Garden Vol. II, Illumination

17. Mothers, in their wisdom, foresee the occult conditions at the birth of a child. The mother's spirit knows how the enemy tries to harm the new wayfarer. During

the transitory time of gestation it is easier to send the poison. It is easy to stir the mother's anger and to fill the home with the dust of discontent.

Mothers try wisely to direct their eyes toward the images of saints or to be comforted through the beauty of nature.

25. Even a simple housewife will say, "Do not soil the steps, or else you will have to clean them of your traces."

125. In the day of woman's humiliation one may trace the appearance of the Divine Mother...

In the future equilibrium of spirit and matter a clear vision may be obtained. But now only fragments are to be seen. That is why the ancients guarded this natural telescope so cautiously. The most powerful telescopes were women, and the first requisite for their protection was quietude.

136. The lofty mission of women must be performed by the woman. And in the Temple of the Mother of the World should abide the woman.

The manifestation of the Mother of the World will create the unity of women. The task now is to create a spiritually sovereign position for the woman. And the transmission to woman of direct communion with the Highest Forces is necessary as a psychological impetus. Of course, through the new religion will come the necessary respect.

138. Urusvati. It is time to say that this is the name We have given to the star which is irresistibly approaching the Earth. Since long ago it has been the symbol of the Mother of the World, and the Epoch of the Mother of the World must begin at the time of Her star's unprecedented approach to the Earth. The Great Epoch is begin-

ning, because the spirit understanding is linked with the Mother of the World. Even to those who know the date it is marvelous to behold the physical approach of the predestined. The approach of this very great Epoch is important; it will substantially change the life of the Earth. A Great Epoch! I rejoice so much, seeing how the new rays are piercing the thickness of the Earth. Even though in the beginning they are hard to bear, yet their emanation induces new elements, so needed for the impetus. New rays are reaching the Earth for the first time since its formation.

Today is the beginning of the feminine awakening. A new wave has reached Earth today, and new hearths have become alight; for the substance of the rays penetrates deeply.

It is joyous to feel the approach of the New Epoch.

140. This is the story of Mary Magdalene:

You know my way of life, how by night people knew us and by day shunned us. So with Christ.

By night they came and by day they averted their faces. I thought: "Here am I, the lowest, and by sunlight people are ashamed of me. But He also, the most Exalted Prophet, is avoided by day. Thus, the lowest and the loftiest are equally avoided."

And so I decided to find Him by day, and to stretch out my hand to Him. I donned my best attire and my necklace from Smyrna, and perfumed my hair. And so I went, to say to people: "Here by daylight are met the lowest and the highest—equally avoided by you."

And when I saw Him, seated among the fishermen and covered with a sackcloth, I remained on the opposite side and could not approach. Between us people passed, equally avoiding us. Thus my life was determined. Because He said to His most beloved disciple: "Take this pinch of dust and bring it to this woman, that she may exchange it for her necklace. Verily in these ashes is more life than in her stones; because from ashes I may create stones but from stones only dust."

The rest you already know. He did not condemn me. He but weighed my chains and the chains of shame crumbled as dust. He decided simply. Never did He hesitate to send the simplest object which determined one's entire life. He touched these sendings as though bathing them in spirit. His path was empty; because people, after receiving His gifts, hastily departed. And wishing to lay on His Hands, He found all empty. When He was already condemned, the furies of shame rushed behind Him and mockingly brandished their branches. The price of the robber was worthy of the crowd.

Verily He cleft asunder the chains because He bestowed knowledge without accepting reward.

150. The Mother of the World appears as a symbol of the Feminine Origin in the New Epoch, and the Masculine Origin voluntarily returns the treasure of the World to the Feminine Origin. Amazons were the embodiment of the strength of the Feminine Principle, and now it is necessary to show the aspect of spiritual perfection of woman.

181. Verily, majestic is the picture of the ocean of the spirit! The sound of the call drones and rings out, and they who have accepted the weapon of the spirit are striving toward the Altar, because the daughter of the world has completed her spiritual raiment.

Onward to battle! battle! battle!

"I hear the call and bow my head before the Command of the Blessed Lord."

192. Afterwards Mary came out of the house and, seeing Christ, said: "Teacher, share our evening meal."

Christ answered: "The gift of the heart glows in the darkness."

204. In ancient cults there was a period called "the condition of opened treasures," when the priestess was already abiding on the eighth floor, entrance to which was prohibited, and the stairs were covered with the skins of leopards in order that no sound might penetrate. This state of "opened treasures" was so reverenced that the violation of the repose was punished as a religious offense.

Everything inharmonious is especially harmful; therefore, a thunderclap is less dangerous than the scream of a newborn. This simple truth was never written down. It is absolutely impossible theoretically to draw a demarcation line of harmony, because the tonality of the accord of spirituality is an individual one.

The ancients knew that the "treasures" are unrepeatable, and took measures against accidents. During the opening of the treasures the Elder of the Temple observed which of a gamut of sounds had the greatest effect. Each sound was accompanied by a definite color—thus were the conditions for each case determined.

218. I wish to recall the cult of the high priestesses. There was one group which was brought into an exalted state by means of chemical preparations; another by way of magnetic currents and there were also low grades of conjurations and mechanical whirlings. Then began the inward concentration on the threshold of sleep or the

concentration upon a brilliant object. The knowledge which came from within, without any apparent conditions, was considered the highest.

230. During the Mystery rites the priestesses were so deeply enwrapped in an almost invisible veil that they ceased to hear and to see, as if the thread of existence had been severed. It was a kind of purification, in an atmosphere full of turmoil.

304. I have already told you about the inner understanding of languages. Write down this legend:

It was once proclaimed that a certain high priestess could understand any language through the inner consciousness, and wonderful results followed. Envoys from far-off lands spoke to her in their own language and she understood them. Thus there was created a legend about the eternal language.

But crowds of people wished to be convinced about it. Many foreigners were brought forward, and the priestess was led down from the eighth floor in spite of her protests. But nothing was manifested for the people, and the strangers reiterated in vain their speeches.

Thus was ruined one of the best possibilities. Yet it would be possible to put this into practice by studying the quality of aura, because this is the bridge of both bliss and contagion.

The ability to understand even one's own native tongue depends not upon the ear but on the contact with other centers through the aura. Therefore, it is better to say, "I have understood," than to say, "I have heard."

Therefore, as to the question of aura, its color is not so important as is its inner intensity.

305. My Hand will not tire to lead, but you do have to

walk, each one with full strength. It is correct to apply one's strength to the difficult, because everything easy is incommensurate with the future.

What does a mother say to her son upon his leaving for war? "Know how to defend thyself." Thus, My warriors also must understand how to fight single-handed.

The chain of the circle may facilitate, but resourcefulness is tested when one is left to oneself.

344. Can Our Community intervene in the affairs of the world and render active assistance? . . . Our envoy once urged a queen to act more in accord with the laws of the time.

355. The spark of the blow gives birth to achievement. Of course, that achievement is preferable which grows consciously, when all one's being knows that the Teacher of Light does exist.

We knew a little girl in whom this knowledge immutably flashed out. Even sickness could not destroy this spirit-knowledge. Its forms were refracted, but the essence remained steadfast.

Thus, extend the essence into Infinity.

359. Astral guests crowd into the midst of life without attention being paid to them. Of course, it is not always easy for them to reach different people, and then one's earthly visitors serve as their mediators. Communication encounters difficulty, but the emanations of auras left by visitors or servants constitute a bridge for the invisible guests. The merit of these is very diverse—from the touch of a butterfly to the jaws of a tiger. Therefore, it is more practical to admit fewer people into your sleeping chambers and your workroom, if your own aura is already sufficiently steady.

Especially dangerous are the educators of children who come in with most horrible companions. The best sendings are often paralyzed by the presence of children's nursemaids and nurses. Therefore, self-activity is always useful. And again it is necessary to pay attention to secretaries, as they have ruined so many affairs.

Do things for yourself, and you may rest tranquil as to the quality of your own emanations.

New Era Community

72. The Community, as Fellowship, can unprecedentedly accelerate the evolution of the planet and give new possibilities of intercourse with the forces of matter. It must not be thought that community and the conquest of matter are found on different planes. One channel, one banner—Maitreya, Mother, Matter!

78. Mother and Teacher—these two concepts must be safeguarded in each book. The light of greatness is not to be extinguished.

95. Once a woman stopped between images of the Blessed Buddha and Maitreya, not knowing to Whom to offer her reverence. And the image of the Blessed Buddha uttered these words: "According to My Covenant, revere the future. Standing in defense of the past, direct your gaze toward the dawn."

102. It is necessary to guide the education of a people from the initial instruction of children, from as early an age as possible. The earlier, the better. You may be sure that overfatigue of the brain occurs only from awkwardness. The mother approaching the cradle of her child utters the first formula of instruction: "You can do everything." Prohibitions are not needed; even the

harmful should not be prohibited. It is better instead to turn the attention simply to the more useful and the more attractive. That tutorage will be best which can enhance the attractiveness of the good. Besides, it is not necessary to mutilate beautiful Images for the sake of an imagined childish non-understanding; do not humiliate the children. Firmly remember that true science is always appealing, brief, precise and beautiful. It is necessary that families possess at least an embryo of understanding of education. After the age of seven years much has been already lost. Usually after the age of three years the organism is full of receptivity. During the first step the hand of the guide must already turn the attention to, and indicate, the far-off worlds. Infinity must be sensed by the young eye. Precisely, the eye must become accustomed to admitting Infinity.

It is also necessary that the word express the precise thought. One must expel falsehood, coarseness and mockery. Treason, even in embryo, is inadmissible. Work "as grown-ups" is to be encouraged. After its third year the consciousness easily grasps the idea of the community. What a mistake to think that one must give a child its own things! A child can easily understand that things may be held in common.

The assertion "I can do anything" is not idle boasting but only the realization of an apparatus.

The most wretched being can find the current to Infinity; for each labor of quality opens the locks.

106. When the family does not know how, let the school teach cleanliness in all ways of life. Dirt comes not from poverty but from ignorance. Cleanliness in life is the gateway to purity of the heart. Who then is

unwilling that people be pure? One should equip schools in such a way that they will be conservatories for the adornment of life. Each object can be considered from the standpoint of love. Each thing must be made a participant in the happy life. Cooperation will help to find a way for each household. Where one person alone does not find the solution, there the community will be of assistance. Not prizefighters but creators will be the pride of the country.

107. The school must not only instil a love for the book but teach how to read—and the latter is not easier than the former. It is necessary to know how to concentrate thought in order to penetrate into a book. Not the eye but the brain and the heart do the reading. The book does not occupy a place of honor in many homes. It is the duty of the community to affirm the book as a friend of the home. The cooperative, first of all, has a bookshelf whose contents are very extensive. There will be accounts of the treasures of the motherland and of her links with the world. The heroes, the creators and the toilers will be revealed; and the concepts of honor, duty, and obligation to one's neighbor, as well as mercy will be affirmed. There will be many examples prompting learning and discoveries.

274. Can there be in the community associations of women, men, and children? Assuredly there can. True associations can be formed following many categories— of age, sex, occupation, and of thought. It is necessary that such branches grow healthy; and not only should they not impede the strivings of people, but they should help each other—and this assistance should be voluntary. One should contribute to the success of each sensible act

of unification. Indeed, when cooperations are of varied nature, then blossoming becomes especially possible. We do not put on shackles, but broaden the horizon. Let children take up the most introspective problems. Let women carry aloft the ordained Banner. Let men give Us joy by constructing the City. Thus, above the transitory will stand out the signs of Eternity.

Agni Yoga

5. The inflation of the blood vessels is characteristic of the development of consciousness, and by technical means must this process be protected from the effect of the sun's pressure upon the solar plexus.

Let us not forget how the priestesses of antiquity were shielded from the sun. They wore breastplates of lithium, covered with wax, the melting of which indicated the danger line of temperature.

Besides immersing the hands in water, immersing of the feet is permitted. Cold baths may be as harmful as the sun rays.

10. When a child plays with a kitten his mother rejoices at his courage, loathe to note that the kitten is still blind.

30. When we meet a woman bearing water, do we know whose thirst she will quench?

121. "Sisters and brothers, one may labor incessantly; and wings grow in the flutter of days and nights."

427. Only goal-fitted simplification can bring dignity to life and safeguard the natural resources. One cannot destroy all the accumulations of cosmic efforts, expecting light-mindedly some undeserved energy!

One has to prepare oneself for each new energy. Every

mother thinks about the future child. It is impossible not to think about the energy which is within us! One has to think about the inalienable possibility.

457. One can notice in children strange and furtive looks as if they see something inexplicable. However, they sometimes speak of a fire, of stars or sparks. Of course, nurses consider it sickness or nonsense, but attention must be paid to just such children. As is known, younger children easily see astral images and, furthermore, especially sensitive ones see the fires of space. Such organisms should be carefully observed from their early days. Be assured that in them lie the possibilities of Agni Yoga; and if placed in pure surroundings they will offer exemplary possibilities. Chiefly, they should not be impeded and frightened.

We have spoken sufficiently about the need of Agni Yoga, and of course the sensitive organisms should be prepared not for the onlookers but for life, as the beholders of the predestined path.

For the mother these observations are not difficult; one has only to know what and why one is observing. I am not speaking about harmful indulgence, without correct evaluation. The observer weighs these abilities unnoticeably, leaving, as it were, casual impressions of guidance. One may notice how joyously the eyes of a child open when its movements and exclamations about that which is sacred are carefully supported. Derision is the worst educator. Sensitiveness is the degree of culture. One cannot make Agni Yogis but can only open the path for them, as the cosmic manifestation does not admit any forcing. But where the flower of fire is ready to blossom, do not hinder.

554. Verily, manifold and intricate as the most delicate design are the manifestations of psychic energy. Not reason but the straight-knowledge of the Chalice can discern them. As a mother knows of the agitation of the child, so does the fire of the Chalice illumine the disturbance of the currents. One may suggest to humanity to ponder as to why the future development puts forward the importance of the Chalice.

It is essential that one add the refinement of thought to the perfecting of technique. What beautiful images will be perceptible to that enlightened eye! Man is responsible not only for himself but for the multitude of consciousnesses.

Infinity I

156. It is truly told about the power of love for humanity. Can one love a garden and despise its flowers? Can one worship the power of beauty and not show respect for love? I attest that the Power adorning Our Universe is confirmed as Our Mother of the World—the Feminine Origin! Indeed, one may cite many scientific examples indicative of the creative destiny of woman. Those who deny the evidence of woman's creativeness should reflect that woman gives voluntarily. It does not mean that those who possess the rights are the ones who affirm them. Hence is the woman's path termed one of voluntary giving. Certainly in Cosmos everything is interwoven, but humanity transgresses the laws of the Higher Reason. Truly, the Feminine Origin is most beautiful! Verily, the pinnacle of Be-ness cannot exist without the Feminine Origin. How badly people have

mutilated the great cosmic laws! How far people have departed from Truth!

The one who possesses the full Chalice We call a voluntary giver.

201. It is very difficult to determine the boundaries in Cosmos between the so-called passive and the active. If We say that all forces are active, men will find this declaration a paradox. But a higher consciousness can understand how We perceive all forces of the Origins as active. The differentiation is so bereft of subtlety that it is difficult to convey to people about the principle which dwells in the manifested power of Mulaprakriti. Likewise, the principle of life cannot be asserted without the realization of the Feminine Origin. Like the Cosmos, Mulaprakriti is a universal principle. The Origins cannot be regarded as competitive forces; only unification of the forces creates life. And We, in the higher worlds, manifest a consecrated reverence for the Origin which humanity calls passive. Yes, yes, yes! The higher consciousness knows the Truth and We are ready to proclaim this Truth to humanity; but for this, humanity must ascend the higher step. Yes, yes, yes! When each Lord had to be given to the world by a mother, how may one not revere Thee, Mother of the World! When each Spatial Fire has to be made manifest in a form, how may one not revere Her who gives life! Yes, yes, yes! How then may one not accept as the highest manifestation of the Cosmos the power in the intense symbol of the Mother!

When the Tara was affirmed on Earth, the three rays of the Lords reverberated. These facets of cosmic fires can be seen on the Tara by a sensitive eye. These facets are so powerfully revealed that their radiance melts all discovered obstacles. One may truly say that the Radiant Image will give new understanding.

Infinity II

21. The potential of spirit of Our Brothers comprises in itself energies identical with those of Cosmos. When We strive toward evolution it may be said that the currents of Cosmos bring identical currents. The Fire of Space lives by the same impulse. Indeed We always imply Sisters as well, when speaking of Brothers. The Origins are affirmed as the equilibrium in Cosmos. He who denies the principle of balance affirms imbalance. Cosmic creativeness necessitates the spirit impregnation of one Origin by the other. Thus, the Origins are created in Cosmos for reciprocal creation. The manifestation of reciprocal creation is affirmed as the symbol of Be-ness.

50. In the eternal creativeness of life, the law of Oneness holds. The cosmic creativeness goes forth as a fiery command; a command preordaining fusion; a command preordaining destiny; a command preordaining the replacement of one by another; a command preordaining consummation; a command preordaining immortality; a command preordaining life for each atom; a command preordaining the approach of the new energy; a command preordaining the New Era. Thus is the cosmic creation accomplished by the magnet of life. How then is it possible to split the creation of the Cosmos? How then can those things which belong to one another be separated? How then can those things which verily issue one from another be separated? Indeed, in its saturation Cosmos is strained for the fiery fusion! Only Cosmic

Reason can give to humanity the Image of Oneness. Reason gives to humanity the supreme Image of the creation of the most fiery Heart. Reason assembles in sacredness; therefore, in Cosmos this law is created by life. Where then is the end, when all cosmic manifestations evolve upon two Origins? When a spirit contacts the higher spheres, cosmic creativeness is revealed to it as the law of infinite unity.

When the spirit reaches the highest Oneness, it may be said verily that it draws from the vessel of cosmic joy. Yes, yes, yes!

Hierarchy

2. When We pointed out the urgency of renewing Our Covenants concerning the equilibrium of the Origins, humanity did not accept this assertion and provoked the manifestation of transgression. Thus, one side transgressed against the cosmic balance.

13. Each Lord has His keynote. The Epoch of Maitreya proclaims the Woman. The manifestation of Maitreya is linked with the confirmation of the Mother of the World, in past, present and future. The "Book of Life" is beautiful!

24. The little girl carrying the heavy volume of the Bible in the chambers of luxury appears as a creator of a new world. The little girl who perceived the Teacher of Light under the blue sky is the destroyer of the dungeons of darkness. When the spirit of a small girl could feel the Brothers of Humanity, then the name of this spirit is a light-bearing sword. When, since childhood, the spirit could sense that the Brothers of Humanity regenerate that which exists, then this spirit holds the light-bearing

name. We cherish the spiritual leaders among children! The evidence of realization is the best gift to evolution. The Command of cosmic life is a summons to light-sustaining achievement, and this mission is affirmed only by Light.

31. The realization of goal-fitness is a token of cooperation with Us. How else may one gain an understanding of the Magnets sent to different countries? How else to approach the manifestation of the magnetization of a human consciousness, which in silence attracts the eyes of an entire nation to itself? Thus one can trace how Our commissioned Sisters and Brothers have attracted and revolved around themselves the consciousnesses of entire nations. But for this one must vigilantly understand the value of each step.

82. The Sons of Reason—We proclaim them as Hierarchs upon the Earth. The Daughters of Reason—thus We proclaim them upon the Earth. Those who strive to the evolution of the spirit must follow in the steps of Hierarchy in order to progress. Who then will nurture the spirit of striving disciples? Who then will affirm the path of ascent? Only Daughters and Sons of Reason. In whom are contained the fires of attainment? In the Daughters and Sons of Reason. Thus We proclaim Our Carriers of Fire. Each realization of Our Will proceeds, manifesting the fiery law of Hierarchy. Only the conscious adaptation in life of the law of Hierarchy affirms a correct path. Verily, the space resounds with the affirmation of Hierarchy. Thus the wondrous life is being built. Thus the predestined enters into life. The Sons of Reason, the Daughters of Light, can manifest the power of the Higher Laws only by obedience to the manifested

Hierarchy. Thus Our Hierarchs manifest Our power of Reason and Heart. Thus to the Infinite!

297. People ask why We do not enforce the striving toward evolution. But even a plain nurse tells a child, "Be like a grown-up, find yourself!"

347. Many salt pillars are spread upon the face of the Earth. Not only did Lot's wife turn back to the past, but numberless are those who looked backwards. What did they expect to see in the conflagrant city? Perhaps they wished to bid farewell to the old Temple? Perhaps they looked for their cosy hearth or looked in anticipation of seeing the house of their hated neighbor collapse. Certainly the past chained them for a long time. Thus, one must strive onward for enlightenment and health and for the strength of the future. Thus it should be always; but there come cosmic knots when an impetuous onward motion is urgent. One should not be disconcerted and mourn over the past. Mistakes are even obvious but the caravan does not wait and the very events press onward. We hurry and We summon to hasten. The future is crowded but there is no darkness ahead.

Heart

96. "Sickness rises from sin," say the Scriptures. We say that sickness comes from the imperfections of past and present. One should know how to approach the cure of sickness. To the annoyance of physicians, the process toward perfection is the true prophylactic measure. One may understand that the process toward perfection begins with the heart, and it has not only a spatial but also a confined material meaning. Mothers carry their children close to their hearts as a panacea for calming

them, but usually one is unaware that this holding close to the heart creates a powerful reaction. Thus, also in the Subtle World We gather people close to the heart for strengthening and for cure. Of course the heart loses a great deal of energy through such strong application. But then, more than once has the heart of the mother been represented as transfixed by swords and arrows, a symbol of the acceptance into the heart of all manifested pains.

Not only in developed sicknesses, but at their inception, is the cure through the heart especially potent. At present, this remedy is almost forgotten, but it is no less powerful than a blood transfusion, because through the reaction of the heart is transmitted the finest energy without the unpleasant low mixture of blood. When one thinks about the process of perfecting, one must not forget solicitude for the giving heart.

106. Why are women often awakened to the Subtle World? Because the work of the heart is much subtler and thus transcendentalism appears easier for them. Verily, the Era of the Mother of the World is based upon the realization of the heart. It is precisely woman alone who can solve the problem of the two worlds. Thus one may call woman to the understanding through the heart. That will also be useful primarily because the quality of the heart is eternal. Already there are many heroic deeds among women, but now instead of the holocaust woman has been accorded the flame of the heart. Let us not forget that for each important achievement the Feminine Principle is essential as a foundation and essence. The heart cannot open to the Subtle World if it is not understood through a special achievement.

239. If a mother does not listen patiently to the first wishes of her baby, she is not a mother. If the Teacher does not show patience to the first steps of a disciple, he is not a Teacher... Patience is the gem of the Crown. It testifies to the approach to Infinity.

284. A simple dairymaid, while she churns her butter, already knows the secret of the formation of the world. She also knows that one cannot make butter out of water. She will say that one can churn milk or an egg; thus she already knows the matter which contains psychic energy. But precisely this condition will not seem convincing to the scientists. The dairymaid also knows how useful is a spiral rotation, but to some this condition will seem a prejudice. Never mind, become angered but think of the surroundings; and transfer the physical laws to your own existence! Only thus wilt thou survive through Armageddon! It would of course be an error to forget the application of the heart as the counterbalance of all confusion.

408. The education of the heart must begin when one is two years of age. First of all, one may advise mother's milk or goat's milk—but the hired wet nurse is a hideous practice. Besides, the mother's milk is often more digestible and already contains particles of the heart energy. But until now this was not taken into consideration; even the simplest people feel more the truth than the cold dogmatists.

453. Verily, nothing is duplicated in the Universe, but the most individual still remains the heart of man. But who can measure the abyss? And who will undertake the task to explain and to reiterate to peoples about the heart? Not lawyers, nor physicians, nor warriors, nor

priests, but the Sisters of the Great Mountain will undertake the solemn duty of laying a hand upon the aching heart, designating with the other hand the unlimited Bliss. Who, then, will know how to understand the solemnity of Love which unites the silver thread with the citadel of the Highest Heart? Therefore We send the Sisters to an achievement of the Heart. It is impossible to manifest the infiniteness of the Highest Heart in the comprehension of an unmanifest consciousness. But you must already be successful in the absorption of solemnity. You must build up solicitude not to violate solemnity by anything petty and lacking in co-measurement. In such a measure shall the Sisters of the Mountain progress in Service. Thus, they will protect the hearts of people from infamy and the stench which is created by darkness.

539. A refined understanding of the needs of the body safeguarded many generations. For instance, one may recollect how cautiously the Egyptians treated the condition of pregnancy. Now people rarely study the tastes or the strange demands of the pregnant one. But formerly, at the inception of pregnancy the temple physician, according to astrological data, defined the necessary mineral and vegetable reactions. Thus the labor itself was eased considerably. But now, instead of wise preliminary measures, people apply coarse narcotics, not desiring to understand that the bond has not yet been severed with the child. The heart of the mother happens at times to be very strained, and each narcotic reacts upon the milk—thus nature is in need of coordination.

549. The family is indicated in all Teachings as the pillar of the entire future. Verily, in addition to all other meanings, the family is the nursery of karmic ties. Thus,

the Teaching would not be complete without affirming the significance of the family. One should regard the family as the hearth of conscious understanding and cooperation. Humanity may meet upon cooperation. And this quality will bring one to the realization of Hierarchy. One should not neglect karmic laws.

Fiery World I

50. Each endeavor may be fulfilled in three ways—either through external muscular exertion, or outwardly through a nerve center, or through the heart's fiery energy. If the first is animal, the second is human, and the third is of the Subtle World. The third form of exertion could be utilized much more frequently if people could consciously apply the concept of the heart and the Fire. But unfortunately this tension arises only in exceptional cases. Naturally, when the mother saves her child, she acts beyond earthly conditions. When the hero dedicates himself to the salvation of mankind, he multiplies his strength tenfold. But this unconscious enflaming rarely occurs. We look after constant growth of the forces through a cognition of the predestined powers.

102. In its timelessness and spacelessness thought belongs to the Subtle World, but also in this structure one must discern still deeper possibilities. Fiery thought penetrates still deeper than the thought of the Subtle World. Therefore fiery thought manifests even more exactly the highest creativeness. With attention, everyone can discern these two stratifications of thought. During the usual trend of thought we often sense that a current, as it were, of a second thought clarifies and

34

intensifies the first. This is not a division of the thought but, on the contrary, a sign that deeper centers have begun an active participation. This flaming process has a special term in Hindu metaphysics, but we will not dwell on it because it will lead to dispute and Western arguments. Such controversies are of no use—all that is needed is a simple reminder of the fact that thought is linked to the World of Fire. Even children exclaim, "It came like a flash!", or "Now I see light!". Thus are termed the moments of correct and instantaneous decisions. One may remember how Mme. Kovalevsky solved mathematical problems. Such fiery condition united with the World of Fire is characteristic. You know that sometimes, above the subtle thoughts, there appear profound thoughts which are difficult to separate from the thoughts of the Subtle World. This is impossible under the present condition of our planet. But even one experience of this dual trend of thought should compel us to realize the division of the worlds.

369. You explained quite correctly the curing of the case of tuberculosis known to you. Many cases of disease, especially among women, come just from the kindling of the centers. But this conflagration may be quenched by urging the consciousness in a useful direction. It is possible that the fiery consciousness had been knocking for a long time, but the sparks of Fohat pierced the region of the Chalice without being utilized. It is in this way that the conflagration starts, and tuberculosis is the most common result of nonassimilation of the Fire. To assimilate in consciousness means already to assimilate physically. This relation of consciousness and body is especially noticeable in the example of Fire, which

causes a quite apparent physical deterioration if not cognized. Therefore, during illnesses, especially those in the nature of colds, it is useful to perform a fiery pranayama. This pranayama is very simple; the usual inhaling through the nose and exhaling through the mouth, the while directing the Prana to the seat of the disease. But for intensification of action one should keep in mind that the Fire of Space is inhaled and the consumed Ur is exhaled. Thus, Fire is again the remedy, and the physician can alleviate the condition of the patient by assuring him how easy it is to attract the basic energy. Fortunately sickness strengthens one's inclination to faith, and a seriously sick patient will accept the truth of Fire more readily.

411. In any home one learns to consider the thoughts of the mistress of the house. Thus, in the midst of daily life, the characteristics of the subtle order are manifested.

502. Is it possible that people do not wish to prepare themselves for the new conditions? Such ignorance recalls the story of the child who had the faculty of seeing in the dark but whose mother asked the physicians to cure the child of this abnormality. The evidences of the work of the fiery centers have become more frequent among people. It is unwise to reject these gifts which will furnish the solution for the immediate future.

561. It is better to go to sleep with a prayer than with a curse. It is better to begin the day with a blessing than to begin in bitterness. It is better to partake of food with a smile than with dread. It is better to enter upon a task with joy than with depression. Thus have spoken all the mothers of the world. Thus have heard all the children of the world. Outside of Yoga, the simple heart knows

what is needed for spiritual progress. One may define it in any terms, but the significance of a joyous and solemn foundation is preserved throughout all the ages. But the Yoga of Fire must strengthen the foundation of ascent. The Agni Yogi, above all, is not a hypochondriac; he summons all those who are strong and joyous of spirit. When joy keeps its glow even under the most difficult circumstances, the Agni Yogi is filled with impregnable strength. There, beyond the most difficult ascent, begins the Fiery World. The manifestation of the Fiery World is immutable. A Yogi knows that nothing can stop him from attaining the Fiery World. Thus the first prayer of a mother and the very splendor of the Fiery World are on the same thread of the heart.

563. Today is a difficult day, therefore I will narrate a story. "A certain demon decided to tempt a pious woman. Dressing himself as a Sadhu, the demon entered the hut of the woman, counting his beads. He asked for shelter, and the woman not only invited him in and set food before him but asked him to pray with her. The demon, the better to succeed, decided to accede to all her requests. They began to pray. Then the woman asked him to tell her about the lives of the Saints, and the demon began to recite like the best of Sadhus. The woman rose to such ecstasy that she sprinkled the entire hut with holy water, and naturally sprinkled some over the demon himself. Then she proposed to the demon that they perform together the pranayama, and gradually she developed such power that the demon finally was unable to leave the hut, and remained to serve the pious woman and to learn the best prayers. A Rishi, passing by the hut, looked in, and, seeing the demon in prayer, joined him in

praise to Brahma. Thus all three sat around the hearth, singing the best prayers. Thus a simple woman, through her devotion, impelled a demon and a Rishi to sing in praise together. But in the Highest Dwelling Place this cooperation occasioned no horror, only smiles. Thus may one compel even a demon to join in prayer."

581. A mother told her son of a great Saint, "Even the grain of sand beneath his foot becomes great." It came to pass that this Saint passed through the village. The boy followed his footsteps, took up a pinch of dust therefrom, sewed it in a bag and wore it around his neck. And as he recited his lessons in school he always held this relic in his hand. The boy thereby was filled with such inspiration that his answers were always remarkable. On leaving the school his teacher praised him and asked him what he had always held in his hand. The boy replied, "Sand from beneath the feet of the Saint who passed through our village." The teacher commented, "This hallowed earth will serve you better than gold." A neighboring shopkeeper, hearing this, said to himself, "What a stupid boy to take only a pinch of this golden earth! I will await the passing of the Holy Man and collect all the sand from beneath his feet. Thus I can obtain the most profitable merchandise." And the shopkeeper sat in his doorway and waited in vain for the coming of the Holy One. But the Holy One never came. Greed is not in kinship with the Fiery World.

649. With great difficulty do people accept instruction outside their usual standard. There are many examples of people's limiting themselves. For instance—a woman has lost husband and children. They are near by, but she will mourn her loss and not move to search for

them. Thus it happens not only on the Earth but also in the Subtle World. One must develop cooperation and persistence here as well as there.

659. One may recall instances from the most ordinary lives when mothers have saved their children and in so doing have withstood the most furious assaults of the elements. A certain substance transformed their forces. Not without reason is it said that metaphysics does not exist; only physics. Physics also teaches that success is created in joy. But what can establish the undaunted joy of the spirit if not the realization of the Fiery World? One must cultivate this realization as a precious flower. The Silvery Lotus glows as a sign of the opening of the Gates of the Future.

Fiery World II

34. A mother sometimes spoke to her son about the meaning of Highest Bliss, and of the eternal link with the Higher Forces. One day the boy very attentively observed a little bird on the window sill, and whispered to his mother—"It also watches me so that I should not say something bad!" Thus may one begin the thought about the great link.

428. Daydreaming must be transformed into disciplined thinking. The ancient sages advised mothers to pass on to their children tales about heroes, and to acquaint them with the best songs about great deeds. Is it possible that humanity nowadays wishes to renounce these wise covenants? The Fiery World is first of all open to heroes—to those who achieve.

Fiery World III

116. The connection between the life of each Servant of Light and the succeeding step reveals a saturated heart-striving. Indeed, people debase the feeling of love and interpret vulgarly the great law. But one must hearken subtly to the great law. Thus, verily, the Yoga of the Heart brings one to the mighty summits of consciousness far more strongly and speedily than does the mind, however refined it may be. Therefore, the great Epoch of Woman will be distinguished by greater refinement of feelings and of consciousness.

170. The ecstasy of Saint Catherine could be made manifest because the Saints lived in a world apart. The pattern of life when such forms were being manifested is so unlike Armageddon! Never before have such spatial battles raged. The tension of all spheres is fiery. On the path to the Fiery World one must be especially conscious of the bond between spheres.

241. It is so indispensable to affirm in the spirit the Feminine Principle. For the Banner of the great Equilibrium of the World has been given to woman to uplift. Thus the time has come when woman must fight for the right that was taken away from her and that she did voluntarily give up. How many powerful records fill space with the attainments of the Feminine Principle! As the Teacher creates through the disciples, so does woman create through the Masculine Principle. Therefore woman flamingly uplifts man. Hence also degeneration, because without true knighthood the spirit cannot rise.

284. So, too, does creativeness proceed according to the spiral, and each vital attraction or repulsion creates its own spiral. That is also why spirals of the Mascu-

line and Feminine Principles proceed in such divergent directions. The Masculine Principle strives for seizure, regardless of the heart of man. The Masculine Principle makes bridges for its achievements by stepping upon hearts and heads. The issue is not brain power, for potentially the Feminine Principle contains the same fires. But the Feminine Principle is in need of freedom for heart expression. When it becomes customary to allow the Feminine Principle to live and develop its potentiality toward regeneration through its feeling of continuous giving, then will the Feminine Principle outdistance the Masculine in all directions.

347. In the future reconstruction of the world, on the higher spheres there will not be access for those who do not understand equilibrium. Long incarnations will be necessary, to study how to create cosmic equilibrium. Indeed, empires have fallen, nations have fallen, countries have been destroyed, all because the greatest question, that of equilibrium, has been reduced to nothing. Therefore it is so important to affirm the significance of the Feminine Principle. Precisely, not in the household measuring scale, but in that of the state. If the planet is retained, then future countries will flourish only through equilibrium. We will even admit a preponderance on the side of the Feminine Principle, because the conflict will be very intense. Indeed, Councils of Ministers will have to include women. Woman, who gives life to a people, must also have a voice in the making of its destiny. Woman must have the right of voice. If woman were accepted, as was ordained, the world would be quite differently impregnated. Thus, only affirmation of the law of Existence can restore the order of man.

478. One who has been chilled by frost brings cold with him. Mothers caution their children, "Do not go near the cold man." One who has been warmed by the sun carries warmth with him. People wish to warm themselves in proximity to him. Is it not the same with the flaming heart which is in communion with the Fiery World? People hasten to the glowing heart to warm themselves and avoid the deadly cold—thus it is in all Existence. Simple and close is the presence of the Higher World, but earthly consciousnesses drive away the ethereal flame with stone blocks.

503. It can be observed that children not only use the words they have heard but introduce words of their own. These will provide clues as to the nature of the inheritance from previous incarnations. One can easily observe the true inherited character and gather evidence of some valuable peculiarities. Even from among the very first expressions of an infant it is possible to form an idea of its inner consciousness. It has not by accident turned its attention to this or that object. Also very significant are the unexpected words uttered in its very infancy. We have already spoken about practically the same thing, but now We are mentioning it from the standpoint of fiery energy. It can be observed that in childhood there is much electricity in the body, relatively the same quantity as in adults, which means that the elements of the fiery body have been fully implanted. The seed of the spirit has been already embedded.

Mothers, remember that children observe and are conscious of more things than you surmise. And many manifestations escape notice: for example, a frequent glowing of the child's body, as well as gestures and occurrences of anger or repose. Erroneously people think that the child's aura is inexpressive. One may see in it not a little of the burden it has brought back.

557. You know that one should speak simply, but people expect the very simplest. One may receive questions such as one is even ashamed to answer. But every mother knows of these questions from her children. The mother conquers her irritation and finds a kind word for the child.

Aum

69. Prayer has no kinship with violence nor constraint. The first prayer of the child should not be ridiculed nor reproved. A boy once prayed: "O Lord, we are ready to help Thee." A passer-by was indignant and called the child presumptuous. But in this way the first feeling of unselfishness was defamed. A little girl prayed about her mother and her cow, and her prayer was ridiculed. But her memory retained, then, only something ludicrous, whereas such solicitude was really touching.

Using the name of God for intimidation is also a great blasphemy. Forbiddance to pray in one's own words is in itself an intrusion into the young consciousness. Perhaps the child remembers something very important and extends its thought upward. Who, then, can intrude to smother such a luminous impulse? The first instruction about prayer will be a direction upon the whole path of life.

70. The surroundings at home likewise impose an imprint on one's whole life. Even the poorest hut may not outrage the spiritual feeling. It should not be presumed that futility of life is not noticed by children. On

the contrary, they feel keenly the structure of all their everyday life, therefore prayer lives best in a clean home.

131. An alarmed child nestles close to its mother's knee, not in supplication but with a feeling of firm support and protection. Likewise, sooner or later, a man in distress turns to the Higher World. He will have nowhere else to go; he may be confused by the advice of uninvited bystanders, hut his heart will be secretly atremble about the Highest.

193. The housewife, who has churned from milk a morsel of butter, has already become initiated into a very important aspect of cosmogony. Thus she can understand the generation of the heavenly bodies. Before beginning her churning the housewife thought about it, and only from a combination of thought and churning was the useful matter produced. Later comes cheese also, already with the embryos of a population. Let us not smile at such a microcosm, the same energy evolves also the systems of worlds. It is necessary only steadfastly to realize the significance of thought, the significance of great energy. Is it not marvelous that the same energy glows in the heart of each man?

199. It has been said—"Many mothers, fathers, wives, sisters and brothers, will be given," yet even such a clear indication does not compel people to reflect as to where this will take place. They do not wish to meditate about earthly lives! The wisest Covenants do not reach ears that are closed.

414. Some await tidings from above, others apply their ears to the ground. Nothing in the Universe can be disregarded.

One should understand the most proximate gifts of

evolution; first—psychic energy; second—the women's movement; third—cooperation. Each of these gifts must be accepted in full measure, not abstractly. We have many times already pointed out the power of psychic energy. Just as insistently should there now be indicated the qualities of the next two distinctions of the age.

415. The Mother of the World! It would seem that in one sounding of these words would be made clear the meaning of the grandeur of the concept, but life shows otherwise.

Poets and singers frequently glorify woman, but governments are unable to recognize simple equality of rights. It will be a shameful page of history which will record that even now equal rights have not yet been established. Woman's bringing-up and education are not on a level with man's and motherhood itself is not protected.

Whoever is first in carrying out such an action of universal import will be proceeding in harmony with evolution.

416. Woman herself must set an example in unity. We know how seldom such harmony is attained. But if the one real motivation be emphasized, then it becomes impossible to remain deaf just by reason of absurd customs. Indeed, many of them have a historical basis, but these obstructions must be destroyed.

By their own hands women of all races and beliefs will help to mold the steps of evolution. There should be no delay!

417. You will encounter two types of opponents of equal rights—one, an admirer of the rule of the harem, who says that age-old customs should not be disturbed;

the other, indignant at the past, will demand supremacy for herself in everything. Both will be remote from evolution.

It is impossible to drag past offenses into the future. It is impossible to preserve also the ossification of an outworn way of life. It is impossible to erect obstacles to free cognition. Affirmation of true equality of rights might better be called full rights. The obligations attending the recognition of full equality will liberate life from coarse customs, from foul speech, from falsehood, from dusty routine. But the new evolution must be begun from childhood if thoughts about it have not flashed out independently.

One may be convinced that at present there are many women who perfectly understand the significance of full rights. They may be relied upon throughout the world.

420. Fullness of rights involves full obligation. Lacking such understanding, full rights will change into arbitrariness. Among women can be found that conscientiousness which will provide the quality of evolution.

Without an innate striving for quality it is impossible to acquire the feeling for perfectionment.

421. Woman may also be judge as well as legal adviser, for injustice will be diminished when the tribunals themselves shall repel the malign principle. Such a distinction must transform the whole way of life.

When I say, "You, women, can comprehend cooperation," I thereby wish to evoke the slumbering fires from the depths of your hearts.

424. Much opposition will be shown to cooperation. Some, through selfishness, will not wish to accept it altogether; others will make use of it for personal gains

but will deny its existence; a third group will unite the concept of cooperation with the overthrow of all order.

There will be a great number of objections; therefore the implantation of collaboration becomes one of the most difficult tasks. An abyss of atavism will appear; the most absurd examples from outworn ages will be adduced; crimes will be enumerated which were the result of dishonest cooperation. Too often obstacles have been set up and the new conditions of life forgotten. The trend toward infatuation by mechanization can be rationally solved by cooperation.

Besides, cooperation must not be limited only to certain aspects of work. Cooperation must be accepted as the foundation of Existence. Only through the broadest cooperation is it possible to find the true relationship of the state to national labor. Otherwise a ruinous indebtedness of the state will increase. The solution of such a problem by means of war will be a sign of barbarism. One must think not about the destruction of nations, but about the improvement of the planet!

When psychic energy occupies its due position, when woman enters as the protectress of culture, when cooperation is made the basis of the structure—then all life will become transformed. Knowledge and creativeness will occupy their manifest position. I say manifest in this sense, that amid remote ages may be found examples of understanding of the significance of science and art.

Cooperation reveals easy paths toward perfection.

425. The questions of self-perfection and of national health are closely connected. Let us summon woman to one and to the other. Both tasks are in need not so much of governmental as of family enjoinment. It is impossible

to command purity of thought, it is even impossible to command purity of speech. It is impossible to command a healthful cleanliness of the home, only enlightenment affirms sanity of spirit and body.

428. Why is the participation of woman so necessary in experiments upon psychic energy? Why is woman's care for flowers so beneficial? Why is woman's touch so curative in cases of illness?

A great number of manifestations can be named wherein precisely woman can lend a special tension of psychic energy. But due attention has not been paid to such special qualities of women. It is rarely understood among physicians why the participation of a woman in operations can be particularly useful. The eternal Feminine Principle has not yet found its just interpretation.

Scholars do not admit that the presence alone of certain people is equal to the strongest apparatus. Experiments are not performed which could note graphically the different reactions which result from different people. Indescribably useful is each experiment with psychic energy.

552. The mother can lay the first foundations of the investigation of psychic energy; even up to birth of the child, the mother will take note of the whole routine of life and of feeding. The character of the future man is already defined in the mother's womb. Already certain peculiarities can be observed which predetermine character, expressed in the desires of the mother herself. However in this case it is necessary to make honest observations. But the capacity of observation itself needs to be cultivated.

Thus again We direct attention not to theories and dogmas, but to experiments and observations.

Brotherhood

100. The collapse of home and family will be not in words and actions but in thoughts. Silently are the foundations undermined. Without noticing it, people themselves foment dissolution. There are not many hearths around which mutual labor is performed in full understanding. Thus, each such home is a step toward Brotherhood.

177. In the simplest examples there can be seen indications regarding forgotten fundamentals. The unaccountable whims of pregnant women will remind us about reincarnation, particularly when the character of the child is traced. Likewise, the latest medicine utilizes the concept of primary energy and points out the nervous origin of many ailments. Immunity is regarded as linked to a condition of the entire nervous system, thus putting forward the significance of the primary energy. How, then, may one not recognize it, when science is paying particular attention to it! Can one deny the basis of immunity? People are especially concerned about their health, yet at the same time they lose sight of the most precious factor. How, then, will thoughts about Brotherhood be created, if the fundamentals of life are left in neglect?

212. Much is said about self-sacrifice and striving toward heaven, but there are examples of lofty self-sacrifice here on Earth. Every mother, under various conditions, in her own way expresses self-sacrifice. But let us be attentive, let us be able to discern the most well

concealed signs of this great feeling, for it is so profound that it shuns expression. Among these beautiful blossoms there is to be found also the means for health improvement. Let us find best words, in order that man should not stumble. In this way also may the understanding of Brotherhood enter life.

Letters of Helena Roerich, 1929-1935, Volume I

1 March 1929. The approaching great epoch is closely connected with the ascendancy of woman. As in the best days of humanity, the future epoch will again offer woman her rightful place alongside her eternal fellow traveler and co-worker, man. You must remember that the grandeur of the Cosmos is built by the dual Origin. Is it possible, therefore, to belittle one Element of It?

All the present and coming miseries and the cosmic cataclysms to a great degree result from the subjugation and abasement of woman. The dreadful decline of morality, the diseases and degeneration of some nations are also the results of the slavish dependence of woman. Woman is deprived of the greatest human privilege—complete participation in creative thought and constructive work. She is deprived not only of equal rights but, in many countries, of equal education with man. She is not allowed to express her abilities in the building of social and government life, of which, by Cosmic Law and Right, she is a full-fledged member. But a woman slave can give to the world slaves only. The proverb "great mother, great son" has a cosmic, scientific foundation. As sons mostly take after their mothers, and daughters after fathers, great is cosmic justice! By humiliating woman, man humiliates himself! This explains today the paucity of man's genius . . .

The woman who strives to knowledge and beauty, who realizes her lofty responsibility, will greatly uplift the whole level of life. There will be no place for disgusting vices which lead to the degeneration and destruction of whole countries.

But in her striving toward education, woman must remember that all educational systems are only the *means* for the development of a *higher* knowledge and culture. The true culture of thought is developed by the culture of *spirit* and *heart*. Only such a combination gives that great *synthesis* without which it is impossible to realize the real grandeur, diversity, and complexity of human life in its cosmic evolution. Therefore, while striving to knowledge, may woman remember the Source of Light and the Leaders of Spirit—those great Minds who, verily, created the consciousness of humanity. In approaching this Source, this leading Principle of Synthesis, humanity will find the way to real evolution.

And woman is the one who should know and proclaim this leading Principle because from the very beginning she was chosen to link the two worlds, visible and invisible. Woman possesses the power of the sacred life energy. The coming epoch brings knowledge about this great omnipresent energy, which is manifested in all immortal creations of human genius . . .

Woman must defend not only her own rights but the right of free thought for the whole of humanity! Through the development of thinking, our abilities will expand. Let us think with the broadest, the purest thoughts. . .

Have you listened to your heart? Does it beat in

rhythm with the Perfect Heart which embraces all of you? Thus, I shall finish with the words about the heart. Let woman affirm this great symbol, which can transfigure the whole of life. Let her strive to transmute the spiritual life of mankind.

The mother, the life-giver, the life-protector— let her become also the Mother, the Leader, the *All*-Giver, the *All*-Receiver. (*Letters Of Helena Roerich*. Vol. I, New York, Agni Yoga Society, 2017, p.13-16)

7 October 1930. The idea of creating the unity of women the world over is more than timely. In the difficult days of world upheavals, of human disunity, of the neglecting of all the higher principles of Being, which are the only true givers of life and which lead to the evolution of the world, there must be heard a voice calling for the resurrection of the spirit and for the bringing of the fire of achievement into all the actions of life. And, of course, this voice must be the voice of woman, who during millenniums has drunk the chalice of suffering and humiliation and has forged her spirit in the greatest patience.

Now, let woman—the Mother of the World—say, "Let there be Light," and let her affirm her fiery achievements. What will this Light be like, and which of her achievements will be the great fiery ones? The banner of spirit will be raised, and upon it will be inscribed "Love, Knowledge and Beauty." Yes, only the heart of the woman, the mother, may gather under this Banner the children of the whole world, without distinctions of sex, race, nationality and religion.

Woman—mother and wife—witness of the development of man's genius, can appreciate the great significance of the culture of thought and knowledge.

Woman—*inspirer of beauty*—knows all the strength, all the synthesizing power of beauty.

Woman—bearer of the sacred power and knowledge of spirit—can indeed become "The Leading One.". .

Knowing that limitation leads to destruction, and that expansion gives creation, let us strive with all our forces toward the expansion of our consciousness, toward the refinement of thought and feeling, so that with the resultant creative fire we can kindle our own hearth.

Let us lay into the foundation of Woman's Unity the striving toward true knowledge, that which knows no human demarcations and limitations. But we may be asked how the true knowledge is to be reached. We shall reply, "This knowledge exists in your spirit, in your heart. Be able to awaken it!"

Striving toward beauty will be the key to it. This knowledge is in each striving toward the General Good. It is indicated in all the Great Teachings which have been given to the world. It is in every manifestation of nature. In forgetting to observe the cosmic manifestations, humanity lost the key to many of the mysteries of Being, and it is just these mysteries that could provide understanding of all the reasons for the present upheavals and miseries. Therefore, while gathering the warriors of spirit, let us direct them toward an awakening of this sacred knowledge. (*Ibid.*, p.43-44)

13 May 1931. The time is not far off when the representatives of the countries will publicly support the cultural projects on a large scale. Let all women and all the younger generation rise in defense of culture against all oppression and persecution; let them guard this life-giving flame with all their power. Nations cannot live without this creative fire. Destruction is inevitable where the Cult-Ur dies away. I want to believe that the powerful "Woman's Unity" will make itself heard and will give a new healthy direction to the mind of youth, will show them the true values and will help them to find the joy of existence by enriching it with a new understanding of each life and each labor. Women—it is your turn to say something new! (*Ibid.*, p.69-70)

17 June 1931. The future League of Culture will manifest its authority and will confirm the balance in this world; but as yet it is too early to talk about it. Even though this League already exists invisibly, first of all the Banner of Peace should be affirmed. People must be imbued with the significance of the value of spiritual creativeness and must learn to respect every manifestation of it. The carriers of spiritual fire will become the true treasures of their countries. First, let women realize all the significance of the raising of the Banner of Peace and Culture, and in powerful union, not only theoretically but practically, let them carry the stones for the building of the New World. Mountains are built from stones. Let us not neglect the smallest stone! (*Ibid.*, p.86)

30 June 1931. The Banner of Peace and the Unity of Women in the name of the New Era of Culture are two of the gigantic historical tasks. Please try to realize how serious is the world situation, and apply all your abilities in order to introduce these salutary ideas. Every step of yours should be thoroughly weighed, and should be in conformity with your great tasks. But never listen to the advice of grey conventionality! All delays will bring even worse wreckage. Uphold the Banner of Culture and the pure affirmations you have received. "Sow widely; it is not right to spill the precious seeds only in your own garden." The most important is not to be afraid of any hostile condemnations because all our offerings for the General Good have not in them a trace of destruction or selfishness! Insist on your rights in the name of the offerings you bring to your own country! (*Ibid.*, p.90)

7 October 1931. Could it be possible that the women's organizations in America will remain indifferent and will not support the Banner of Culture? I do hope that we are not over-estimating their spiritual receptivity. Long before the first conference, in Bruges, I learned about the real value of many modern organizations, and I understood how much one must work in order to awaken the consciousness of the masses to make them understand the true values and cultural creativeness. This can be achieved only by the *persistent and systematic spreading of ideas*, but not by convulsive bursts. Therefore, let us not be discouraged by the attitude of indifference shown by governments and certain groups of civilized society, but let us use all our efforts for destroying superficial thinking among the nearest co-workers, as well as for deepening their understanding of the pressing necessity to fulfil this idea. (*Ibid.*, p.103)

1933. Regarding the League of Culture and the Woman's Unity, do not be disappointed by the slow development. Nothing should be forced. First of all, only a very small group is necessary. Very carefully test the newcomers. It is a great art to know how to talk to people according to their consciousness, to give them no more and no less than they can assimilate at the moment. (*Ibid.*, p.142)

8 February 1934. Apart from the caste system, child marriages are bringing degeneration. It is not unusual to see a nine-year-old girl married to a sixty-year-old man and already a crippled mother of a stillborn child. Yes, there are many wonders in India, but also many terrible things! It is as if this would prove the law: "the brighter the Light, the deeper the darkness." That explains why nowhere else do you meet such spirituality and refinement as here. If this beautiful country could succeed in curing the dreadful scourge which is destroying it, the development of this country would amaze the whole world. There are some signs of revival. The woman of India is awakening and her heart reacts to the suffering of the degraded; therefore, she is destined to revive her country. (*Ibid.*, p.158)

17 April 1934. Of course, the Society for Unity of Women needs the hand of a woman. However, man's collaboration is not undesirable and can be most beneficial. Often, man is a better co-worker, apologist and defender of women's rights than many women.

The statutes about the Unity of Women which you worked out are beautiful, and may God help them materialize, even if only partially. I particularly approve the point regarding equal education for both sexes, or, as you call it, "equal rights."

This is a very important matter. Equal education will eradicate the harmful superiority toward women and will give a necessary balance in many other respects. Equality of rights for both sexes, as well as for all nations, should be one of the first foundations of each government.

Everything concerning the upbringing and schooling of children is very dear to me, and I shall willingly share my thoughts about it with you.

You mentioned a most painful problem of today's life—the question of the legality of abortion. Of course, there are no two opinions on this subject: abortion is most definitely murder. Therefore, only in cases where the mother's life is in danger should it take place. But it is wrong to think that a woman who is guilty of abortion always attracts low spirits. The karma of the whole family should be taken into consideration. Often we can notice that in a family where one of the children is worthless the other children are not bad. Karma ties groups of people for long, long thousands of years. And often, even a high spirit has not unimpeachable, irreproachable parents. And it is significant that the dark forces are especially against the reincarnation of highly developed spirits, and they try their best to prevent the reincarnations that are dangerous for them. And, once more, it is not the purgatory of the Subtle World that prevents spirits from reincarnating, but only the crime of the parents. There is not a more powerful purgatory than the earthly life, if all the potentialities of the individuality are intensified. It is said in the Teaching, "As the one who hungers longs for food, even so, the spirit that is ready to incarnate longs for the new incarnation." Therefore, one can imagine what suffering the spirit undergoes by reason of artificial prevention. The spirit is connected with the embryo at the moment of conception, and gradually enters the body in the fourth month when the nerve and brain channels are being formed.

Therefore, abortion is permissible only in exceptional cases.

Of course, woman should not only be a giver of physical life; she has her other high duties. And for that purpose there is the most natural abstinence, which can easily be practised and the increase of the family thus regulated. This is quite possible when high interests occupy the head and the heart. Of course, I expect plenty of opposition; still, I insist on it. No doubt, in the present state of the family it is quite difficult, but already there are such families and they will increase in the future. In remote antiquity, people knew how to regulate their families by the phases of the moon. Later on this was considered black magic, but nowadays even such measures would be better than the dreadful abortions that cripple women and therefore the coming generations. (*Ibid.*, p.164-165)

17 August 1934. And now, regarding the question "In what can the majority of women cooperate?" we must proceed from the fundamental point. Therefore, I would say that they could collaborate in the task of establishing the balance of the world. Verily, the existing state of imbalance threatens humanity as well as the whole planet. How can the world endure when the foundations of life are violated! Much has been said about this in the Teaching, and one can develop the hints that are given. I shall quote several affirmations: "The Banner of the great Equilibrium of the World must be raised by woman. Thus the time has come when woman must fight for rights that were taken from her as well as those she sacrificed voluntarily."

The universal disorganization which we see today,

the threatening degeneration of many countries, is the result of this continuing imbalance through the subservience and oppression of woman. By degrading woman, man degrades himself; and without the revival of true chivalry and gentleness the spirit cannot rise.

It is also said: "As the Teacher creates through his disciples, even so woman creates through the Masculine Principle. Therefore woman uplifts man." Hence, woman must raise herself to such a degree, spiritually, morally and intellectually, that it will enable her to carry man with her. Remember the painting by N.Roerich, "She Who Leads." Thus, woman must occupy the place destined for her. She must become not only an equal cooperator in the management of the whole of life, but also an inspirer. The greatest task is to spiritualize and to restore the health of humanity by filling it with aspiration toward great deeds and beauty. But woman must first of all change herself! Therefore, the call to woman must be primarily the call to self-perfection, for the realization of her dignity and her great destiny and to lay the foundation of Be-ness and for the awakening of the impulse toward creativeness and beauty. It is said: "The Equilibrium of the world cannot be established without true undemanding of the First Causes. . . Therefore, let us be affirmed in consciousness upon the power of Equilibrium, as the stimulus of Existence, of the First Causes, and of Beauty. Hence it is so indispensable to affirm in the spirit the Feminine Principle. . ."

The legend about twin souls has a profound significance. And this law is indicated in the stars. The ancients knew how to read these signs. The key to this was given to the High Initiates. But today such knowledge in the hands of corrupt humanity would bring more misery and calamity than benefit and happiness. Therefore, the Great Teachers are so anxious to awaken spirituality and to broaden the consciousness, as They wish to give humanity the knowledge of the great laws. This is why these laws can be mentioned now only as being within the reach of the science of the future. Nevertheless, it is quite appropriate to mention the existence of these laws, as it is necessary to prepare the thought to work along this line...

Yes, the time has come when woman should be prepared to participate in the burdens and leadership of government. Woman, the life-giver, who lays the first foundations of education, has also the right to create better conditions for those she brings into the world. Her common sense, and especially her heart, will dictate to her many correct decisions. If we take the historical facts and true biographies of many great people, we shall see that often the source of their inspiration and their chief adviser was a woman. Thus, in ancient Egypt the head priestesses often inspired the Hierophants by transmitting to them the will of their Goddess. Thus, they were called the inspirers of the leaders of the people.

The great epoch of Woman is coming. Verily, woman has a two-fold task: to uplift herself and to uplift her eternal companion, man. All the Forces of Light are awaiting this great deed. The Star of the Mother of the World has indicated the great date. All Scriptures are confirming that woman will sever the head of the Dragon. Let the heart of the woman become aflame with this self-sacrificing deed. Let her fearlessly raise the shining but cleaving Sword of the Spirit.

At the destined hour we will call the burning hearts and the hands ready to raise the Chalice of Salvation of the World.

Let every day of our lives be spent in self-sacrificing service to the great task.

The Great Mother is approaching! (*Ibid.*, p.253-257)

16 January 1935. Were it not for the self-sacrifice of the High Spirits, we would be even now in the state of troglodytes. Our earthly humanity owes its accelerated evolution to its Elder Brothers and Sisters, the Great Teachers. (*Ibid.*, p.350)

8 May 1935. The idea of "The Community of the Heroic Sisters" was my dream from an early age! I imagined these women bringing light and joy into the most remote corners and into the hardest conditions of the life of our country. Of course, my dreams grew together with my consciousness, and now I think of all the different aspects of life that could find their reflection in such a Community. Thus, some Sisters could devote themselves to medicine; others to agriculture; others could be teachers or lecturers in the various branches of knowledge and on social problems, expounding them in a way close to the people's understanding. The study of the arts and crafts and the teaching of them would be most important in my Community, together with an investigation into the significance of color, sound and scent, and their influence on man's general condition. The function of the Living Ethics would be to beautify the whole useful movement of these Sisters. Small groups of this Community could be widely scattered, and the Sisters could organize little tours for investigation and observation of those districts which were under their supervision. A whole army of such women workers would be necessary to supply all present needs and to satisfy the spiritual and physical hunger of the people. Schools could be established by the Central Community, as well as universities, laboratories and an institute for research in psychic energy. Furthermore, all sorts of workshops, sanatoria, cooperatives, model farms, etc., could be built up—in short, a whole city of knowledge! The Great Teacher, speaking of these Heroic Sisters, said so beautifully, "Let them endear themselves to people. Let people say, 'A dear one came to our village.' " Indeed, my Sisters would have to learn first of all to be close to the people. I know that it is not at all easy to find selfless heroines; nevertheless, I do not lose hope, as I know that even a small group devoted to this task could work miracles. Now you understand my joy when I find new souls that resound to my innermost thoughts. It seems to me that the coming epoch will attract souls full of aspiration to fulfil the beautiful, active, self-sacrificing deeds. (*Ibid.*, p.411)

31 May 1935. Wrong are the assertions found in books that all religions and teachings discuss the low level of woman. Such discussions as do appear are the distortions and additions made in later times by those holding power through avarice and ignorance. Verily, the Great Founders of religions and teachings are not to be blamed for this crying ignorance. Let us consider how many dishonest and avaricious hands have handled these teachings during thousands of years!

Buddha held woman in the greatest esteem, and stated that she could achieve, as well as man, the highest degrees of Arhatship. Verily, the same fire of spirit, the same monad is aflame in woman as in man; the psychic apparatus of woman is more subtle than that of man. That is why in ancient Egypt the high priestesses of Isis transmitted the orders of the Goddess to the Hierophants, but never vice versa. If our Christian Church has humiliated woman to the extent that during the marriage service the minister proclaims "the wife shall obey her husband," in ancient Egypt it was entirely different because there the wife was the head of the household. Many curious things are still to be revealed. Truly, we dwell in the Maya of our ignorance. This is due not only to a meagerness of tangible proofs and facts, but to the inherited ailments of prejudice and negation. From very early childhood this malady eats into our thinking like a cancer.

True history, and especially true knowledge, will reveal many astonishing pages and real facts. Let us recollect these great words: "It could be said that not a single Covenant has reached us without distortion. Endless are the alterations and distortions which have appeared in the translations of the great writers." How terribly distorted are the works of the first Fathers of Christianity. Let us take, for instance, the great Origen. Do we not have an example of such distortion in the preface to his works written by his disciple? Verily, the deeper we ponder upon the origins of all the Teachings, the more clearly is their oneness and grandeur manifested. Therefore, in our ignorance, let us not accuse the great Founders of the Teachings who assuredly knew about the great law of the Equilibrium of the Elements. In antiquity the last and highest Initiation was connected with this illumination and knowledge. The entire mystery, the whole beauty of Be-ness was revealed to the soul illumined by the highest Light. Even in distorted Hinduism there are preserved some hints of the significance of the Feminine Element. And even up to the present day, the most sacred ritual cannot be performed by a Brahmin without the participation of his wife.

Christ also asserted the equality of the Elements; but dark were the followers of his disciples, and this darkness increased, so to speak, not in arithmetic but in geometric progression.

Likewise, Zoroaster highly esteemed the Feminine Element, and in his Covenants one may find remarkable hints as to the grandeur of Cosmic Love...

Who can tell where woman's rights—rights given to her by Nature—begin and where they end? The same question could be asked about man's rights. Only evolution gives the answer and points out the direction. There is no indication in Nature that woman should be restricted to her hearth! Verily, she is the Mother and Custodian of the World. Hence, there is not a single domain of life where man could rule alone. *It is precisely this domination of the one Element that has created the dark epoch.* Creativeness is given equally to both Elements. In man it is more pronounced at the moment only because woman has been deprived of equal education and has not had the same possibilities for exercising her creative forces on a broad scale. Even today an ignorant belief prevails that the brain of the woman is lighter and smaller than that of the man, and that therefore woman is more stupid, etc. I remember how amazed were the scientists when, after the death of the brilliant writer, Anatole France, his brain was weighed and was found to be amazingly light— almost like a child's brain! Likewise, when some one once said that the more developed is the animal the bigger is its brain, I remember that the Teacher pointed out that some insects are cleverer than animals. Take as an example the ants or the bees. A heavy weight of brain signifies great physical endurance, but not refinement. Entirely different are the signs of great intelligence. The convolutions of the brain have great significance. However, here also, only a partial conclusion may be reached, as very little is known about the mysteries of the inner man. There was another, still more ridiculous, theory of the anthropologists that the bigger the skull is, the more intelligent is the man. Here again, Nature proved the contrary, as it was found that the size of the skull of the island savage is larger than that of the average witty Frenchman. Today, many have come to the conclusion that there are no grounds for considering the mental abilities of woman below those of man.

The dark epoch tried to make out of woman a concubine and a nurse. But if woman stands high as a mother, it is not only as mother in the family, but as Mother and Great Teacher of the consciousness of nations! Thus, as it is said in the Teaching, "Woman, who gives life to people, has the right to govern their destiny. We want to see woman taking part in government, in the councils of ministers, in all constructive activity." But it is said at the same time that ". . . the struggle between the two Elements will he hard, and woman herself will have to recapture her rights which she voluntarily relinquished."

But the violated equilibrium has had such a terrible effect on the life of the whole planet that it is now in danger of destruction! And cosmic justice and goal-fitness once more come to the rescue by bringing forward more and more talented women. In the younger countries destined for evolution, one may observe the way in which woman expresses herself. Thus, in America, there are already women ministers, women diplomats, ambassadors, state governors, directors of the largest firms, aviators, lawyers who win the most complicated cases. Also, a trusted personal secretary of the President is a woman. Indeed, in America women are the main promoters of education and culture. Even most of the "wunderkinder" are to be found among little girls. All these are good omens of the coming epoch. (*Ibid.*, p.420-426)

18 June 1935. Intellect began its development on the physical plane during the fourth root-race of our fourth cycle, when complete immersion into matter took place. But the impetus for its development was given by the Great Spirits, the Sons and Daughters of Wisdom (Elohim) who came from the higher worlds and were incarnated at the end of the third race. Of course, They were of the Divine Dynasty of Spiritual Teachers, of whom accounts are abounding in the most ancient mythology and legends. Precisely, through their incarnations and their direct progeny They transmitted to humanity an organism far more refined, capable of responding to higher vibrations. Likewise, contact with their high fiery auras kindled fires in those who were near Them. Thus, following the current of the natural law of development, humanity, in the majority, is not able to become perfect and have its seven principles or forty-nine fires opened before the seventh race in the seventh cycle...

The Mother of the Universe, or of the manifested Cosmos, can be accepted as one of the Figures of the Holy Trinity. Indeed, there is no religion, except later ecclesiastical Christianity, in which the Feminine Element is not included among the Primates of Be-ness. Thus, the Gnostics also considered the Holy Ghost as a Feminine Element. In the most ancient Teachings, the manifested Trinity of Father, Mother, and Son was considered as an emanation of the highest, eternally hidden Cause; and the latter, in turn, as that of the *Causeless Cause*...

Only the profound ignorance of the Middle Ages could discard the Feminine Element from the construction of all Being. Verily, in their origin both Elements, Male and Female, are united, and one cannot exist without the other. (*Ibid.*, p.445-450)

AGNI YOGA SERIES

Leaves of Morya's Garden I (The Call) 1924

Leaves of Morya's Garden II (Illumination) 1925

New Era Community 1926

Signs of Agni Yoga

Agni Yoga 1929

Infinity I 1930

Infinity II 1930

Hierarchy 1931

Heart 1932

Fiery World I 1933

Fiery World II 1934

Fiery World III 1935

Aum 1936

Brotherhood 1937

Supermundane (in 3 volumes) 1938

Letters of Helena Roerich, Vol. I 1929-1935

Letters of Helena Roerich, Vol. II 1935-1939

AGNI YOGA SOCIETY
www.agniyoga.org

www.ingramcontent.com/pod-product-compliance
Lightning Source LLC
Chambersburg PA
CBHW072156020426
42334CB00018B/2030